OVERCOMING
Panic
Attacks

D1397524

OVERCOMING

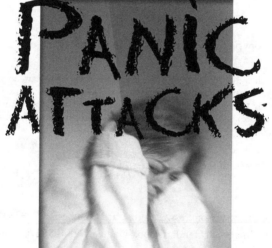

PANIC ATTACKS

by Ray Comfort

Bridge-Logos
Alachua, FL 32615 USA

Bridge-Logos
Alachua, FL 32615 USA

Overcoming Panic Attacks
by Ray Comfort

Copyright ©2005 by Bridge-Logos

Printed in the United States of America.

Library of Congress Catalog Card Number: 2008923296
International Standard Book Number 978-0-88270-014-4

Unless otherwise indicated, Scripture quotations are from
the *Holy Bible: King James Version.*

G163.319.B.m802.35250

Contents

Introduction

Hi, Ray. What are you doing?" The voice on the phone was a familiar one. It was that of Todd Friel, the popular Christian talk show host. But he was *whispering*, which was a little strange for Todd. He's kind of loud.

I whispered back, "I am waiting to be interviewed on a radio program." We had been through this tongue-in-cheek scenario many times. When Todd was short of a guest, he would often call me out of the blue and say, "What are you doing?" When I answered that I was waiting to be interviewed, he would reply "Good. You're on in eight seconds."

Todd was not only sharp; he was funny. He had spent much of his life making his living as a very successful stand-up comedian. Now he devoted himself to teaching Christians how to share their faith. A few years earlier, he had latched onto the teaching on the importance of using God's Law (the Ten Commandments) to reason with the world, and he had run with it with a passion. Mr. Sharp was on the cutting edge of Christian radio. He would call random numbers and say, "Hello. I'm Todd Friel from KKMS. You are live on the radio, so don't swear. May I ask you some questions about your belief in God?"

It was *fascinating* radio. More than often people would open up with him and share their convictions. If they hung up, it was fine. It didn't faze Todd. He would say something witty and then call another number. If they were antagonistic, that was good also. It not only made interesting radio, but it was educational for the listeners because it showed them how they could deal with antagonistic people. If the person was open to the things of God, he would go through the Commandments, and then ask if he may call back the following week and talk further with them about spiritual matters. Most would give permission to do so. The next week, there were listeners. Lots of them. The unscripted don't-know-what's-going-to-happen-next "Talk the Walk" had a huge following.

The day before the whispering call, Todd had phoned me and said that he was going to preach open-air style at the local university. Kirk Cameron and I had gone to the same university six months earlier and showed how to gather a crowed and what to say to hold them. The hardest thing about preaching the Gospel in an open-air situation is pulling a crowd together. It is easier to pull a shark's tooth at dinnertime than it is to get sinners to come and hear how they have offended God. That was understandable. So, for years I would give away money to attract folks. I would ask trivia questions and when someone got one right, I would have the Christians give loud applause and give the person a dollar reward for the right answer. The loud applause usually attracted attention. Or I would put a dummy on the ground, cover it with a sheet, and talk about death. That often attracted attention. Death does that. Fortunately, with Kirk by my side, we had the great advantage of his celebrity. We also had "rent-a-crowd" that evening. About 200 of Todd's faithful following had braved a cold and wet Minneapolis night to join us, and a crowd draws a crowd.

I opened, and then Kirk and I tag-teamed for about an hour. It was a very encouraging night. It was so encouraging that it had inspired Todd to go it alone, *live* on the radio, of course. He didn't have a dummy, nor did he have Kirk, so his phone call that day was to get some final instructions before the open air. I said that an important key was to keep one eye on the Cross. He was there to preach Christ crucified, and if he spoke on the subject of evolution (which he intended to do), it would be very easy to get sidetracked, and almost forget to preach the Cross.

Todd was Mr. Confidence. He was never short of a word. After all, as a stand-up comedian, he had spoken in front of audiences 1,500 times. He had learned to conquer his fears. He had mastered the art of the control of his mind and control of his audience. Yet, he said that the very thought of standing up and preaching the Gospel to unsaved people terrified him. This was a fear that was rational in one sense. It was different than the irrational terror of a panic attack.

The thought of being rejected as a human being, or experiencing the humiliation of drying up in public is a fearful thought for most of us. We can identify with that sort of fear. I could. The first time I ever spoke in public to non-Christians, I was terrified.

So here I now was, listening to a whispering Todd Friel, asking what I was doing. He then said, "Ray, I preached open-air for two to three hours. What happens if you preach open air for three hours?" I said, "You lose your voice. I forgot to tell you that." He whispered back, "Yes, you do. I have a three-hour talk show to do … and I have no voice. You are live on radio, so don't swear. You have a lot of sermons. Preach to us. Help me fill in seven minutes."

Then there was silence. Dead silence. The consummate, ever-talking Gatling-gun of Christian radio, the never-short-of-a-word live standup comedian was dead serious. He had no voice, and he wanted me to fill in for him.

Todd had put the ball in my court, and he was hoping that I would serve him. I mumbled, "I just finished writing a book called, *Overcoming Panic Attacks*—practical advice for those suffering from panic attacks and irrational fear. In my mind I was thinking, "I don't want to get into this. I'm not ready. I'm not an 'expert' on panic attacks. What am I going to say?"

Todd whispered, "Tell me about it. What is a panic attack?" His return was a short ball with a spin on it. I would just have to give it my best shot. Fortunately, the material was fresh in my mind, so for the next seven minutes, I told the listeners about my initial attack and how it left me devastated. He pressed me for advice to listeners who might be sufferers. I told him how I didn't really want to get into that, because it would sound a little silly to those who didn't understand. Only those who have experienced the power of fear can know what it's like. He pressed me further. So, I talked about controlling breathing during an attack. He then opened up the phone lines. There was an immediate response. One man even had a panic attack while he was talking to me live on the radio. My heart went out to him.

Typically, with the colorful host, I suddenly became "Doctor Comfort," and as such, I was dealing out advice on the complex issue of panic attacks. My diagnosis was a simple one. I believed that there were many people who were suffering in silence from the plague of fear. The prognosis was very positive. There *was* hope for the hopeless. But it didn't come in the form of a quick fix pill. All I could offer were a few practical things to help along the way. But I did have a glorious consolation—a wonderful comfort besides the practical advice. The consolation was in the Gospel. It was the knowledge that if those poor folks, who were cursed with panic attacks, would simply trust themselves to God through the Savior, they then would become *rich* folks, who were most blessed. The poor in spirit would be rich in Heaven, and Jesus said that because of that, they were blessed.[1] If their terrible fears caused them to let go of the things of this world, and hold on to the Kingdom of God, they were blessed.

The seven minutes stretched into forty minutes, during which time a woman called who had been listening to Todd for three weeks. She was an unbeliever who, over those three weeks, had opened her heart to the truth. But she had one earnest question. "Go ahead, ask Mr. Comfort."

The listener asked, "What's the difference between Jesus Christ and other great leaders who had died for what they believed in?" It was a good question. What *was* the difference? I said that in the beginning, when God first made man and woman, sin entered the world, and the Bible says that death came by sin. And so, death passed on to all of humanity, because we had all sinned.[2] We would die because we had violated God's Law.

"But," I said, "this same Judge, who proclaimed the death sentence upon all humanity, is rich in mercy. He doesn't want us to perish, and He became a human being in Jesus Christ to solve our terrible dilemma. Jesus was God manifest in human form. This wasn't just a great leader. It was God in Christ ... a perfect man who came to this earth to suffer and die on the Cross to satisfy a perfect Law that demanded perfection. God was manifest in the flesh.[3] He suffered so that our death sentence could be commuted. He paid our fine in His life's blood, so that we could live. Then He rose from the dead and defeated death forever, and all who repent and trust in Him receive remission of sins. God grants them the gift of everlasting life."

The next day I received an email. It said, "We have a list of names of people who called pleading for the book … I think you are onto something again, Mr. Comfort. Todd."

Ray Comfort

END NOTES

1 See Matthew 5:3
2 See Romans 5:12
3 See 1 Timothy 3:16 KJV.

The Splinter

The pastor on the other end of the phone had a deep concern in his voice as he told me that his 60-year-old mom was having panic attacks. His concern was that he had no idea what he could do to help her. The attacks began when a doctor gave her drugs five years earlier. Reaction to the drugs caused them. When she stopped taking them, the panic left.

However, two months before the pastor's phone call, she had been lifting boxes while cleaning her home, and suddenly had a panic attack that left her devastated. In that two months, she had hardly slept or even eaten, had lost thirty pounds, and was entertaining suicidal thoughts.

The Terrifying Anatomy of a Panic Attack
If you are reading this book because someone you care about is having panic attacks, I want

to give you some insight as to what they are about. Lend me your imagination.

You are asleep in bed, when suddenly a creak of the floor causes you to open your eyes in the semi-dark room. Towering over you stands the ugly sight of a huge man, wearing a stocking over his face. He has a gun pointed at your head. Suddenly, your heart races with fear. Your mouth becomes dry. Terror paralyzes you. You can see demons in his eyes. His evil lips smile in delight at having a human being under his power. Time stands still. Your racing heart is taking too much blood into your brain, feeding it an oversupply, making your mind go blank. This inability to respond, even mentally, brings a panic that causes your breathing to become erratic. The over-action of the heart also speedily lifts your body temperature to a point where cold sweat is forming on your brow, back, and legs.

With malicious intent, the intruder slowly moves the gun to the temple of your moistened brow. You can feel its cold barrel against your warm skin. The reality of what is happening tells you that this is no mere nightmare.

Adrenaline is being pumped throughout your body. Your mind is instinctively screaming *Run!* It's the flight or fight syndrome. Yet, you dare not fight. You know that if you move, you are dead. With both hands on the gun, the cruel intruder slowly cocks the weapon. You see his white teeth grit in perverted glee. *You are going to die a horrible death!* Unspeakable terror grips your mind. Perspiration pours out of your flesh. Your mouth is totally dry. It's as though your heart is pounding through your chest. Your breath seems to have drained from your lungs and you can feel your eyes bulge with overwhelming dread ...

That's what an attack of irrational fear feels like. There is no intruder, no gun, and no threat of death. Yet, there are those same, very real, worse-than-nightmarish symptoms.

Welcome to the world of panic attacks. They break into a happy life and steal the joy of living. If you are having panic attacks or irrational fears, you are not alone. Millions in the United States suffer from them. Still, you feel alone. You think that you are losing your mind. You feel hopeless. But there are certain things that you can do to fight them. I know, because in the mid-1980s, my life was put on hold because of the terror of panic attacks. I will share the details with you a little later in this book and tell you what I did to stop them. Before I do, I have to tell you a story.

Without Minimizing its Seriousness, Getting a Panic Attack into Proper Perspective

A child was once running through a wooded area when he fell onto a sharp stick and cut his jugular vein. His father immediately scooped him up, held his thumb on the child's bleeding neck, and rushed him to a nearby hospital.

A short time later, the father, still carrying his son, burst into the local hospital. As a surgeon approached them, the small boy lifted his hand to the surgeon. When he fell, a tiny splinter penetrated his thumb, and he wanted the surgeon to take it out. Of course, the good doctor ignored the child's plea, and immediately began work to stop the bleeding and repair the life-threatening injury to the child's neck.

In our ignorance, we often come to God with things that seem important to us. We hold our splintered thumbs up to God, and fail to see that there is something else, which is truly life-threatening. Our life's blood is gushing from our necks, but we have little concern. Let me tell you what that life-threatening problem is; then we will look at what is still important to you, the "splinter" of panic attacks.

As we look at this issue, you may be tempted to push away the surgeon's hand and hold up your thumb, but please don't do that. What I am going to say is truly life-threatening, and once you see that, it will bring your problem into perspective.

Did you know that in the United States more than 90 percent of the population believes in the existence of God? Even more amazing is the fact that 60 percent of the population believes in a literal Heaven and a literal Hell. The "Hell" part (for those who believe in a God who is all-loving) seems a little hard to reconcile, until we give the subject some serious thought. Ask yourself if you believe that God is good. Most people think He is. Should He then punish a man who viciously molests and murders a little girl? Let's personalize it. Let's say it's *your* cute little eight year-old or your young sister. He rapes her, then calmly strangles her to death, and leaves her tiny body on the side of the road, burned beyond recognition.

Should God have any desire that the man is brought to justice? Humanity does. We have court systems that punish such criminals. How much more should God care? If He didn't care, then we are saying that He has less sense of justice than sinful man. Of course, God should have a desire to see that justice is served. It's logical that if He is good, then He should punish vicious murderers. So divine justice makes sense, and the Bible says that His place of punishment for crime is a "prison" called Hell.

Here's another question. Is God good enough to make sure that a brutal rapist gets justice? Of course. Because He has concern for justice (punishment for crime), God is good; He is not evil like a corrupt judge who turns his head when he sees injustice. C. S. Lewis said, "There is no doctrine which I would more willingly remove from Christianity than the doctrine of Hell, if it lay in my power. But it has the full support of Scripture and, especially, of our Lord's own words; it has always been held by the Christian Church, and it has the support of reason."

Notice his last words. He said that the existence of Hell "has the support of reason." In other words, when you think about it, its existence is reasonable. It makes sense.

Here now is the bottom line. The Bible says that God is so good that He's not going to stop at rapists and murderers, but He will also punish adulterers, thieves, liars, fornicators (those who have had sex out of marriage), and blasphemers. He will punish sin right down to our thoughts. How will you do on that Day of Judgment? Do you think that you will be punished? Have you broken any of the Ten Commandments? Is God first in your life? Have you made a god to suit yourself? Have you ever used God's holy name in vain? Have you kept the Sabbath holy? Have you always honored your parents implicitly? Have you hated anyone? Then the Bible says you are a murderer. Have you had sex out of marriage? Then you are a fornicator and cannot enter Heaven. Jesus said, "Whoever looks upon a woman to lust after her has committed adultery with her in his heart." Have you ever lusted? Have you ever stolen something (irrespective of its value)? Then you are a thief. If you have told just one lie (even if you call it "white"), you are a liar and cannot enter the Kingdom of God. Listen to your conscience. God's Law leaves you guilty. On Judgment Day, if you are found to be guilty, you will end up in Hell forever. There's your life-threatening problem. That dilemma dwarfs your other problems.

But listen to this. Jesus said, "Only the sick need a physician." He has made provision for you to have a life-saving operation. Although we are guilty of violating God's Law, Jesus paid our fine on the Cross 2,000 years ago. We can be forgiven. The Bible says, "God commended His love towards us, in that, while we were yet sinners, Christ died for us." Then Jesus rose from the dead, and defeated the power of the grave. We can be justified (made right with God) through simple faith (trust in Jesus). If you repent and trust in the Savior, God will forgive your sins and grant you everlasting life. So, what are you waiting for? Confess your sins to God right now. Put this book down and be honest before God. Think of your past sins, and tell Him you are sorry, and that you will turn from all sin. Then put your faith in Jesus Christ. Trust Him as you would trust a parachute to save you. It's more than just an intellectual belief. It is trusting Him with your eternal salvation. Then read the Bible daily and obey what you read (see John 14:21). If you are not sure how to pray, open your Bible at Psalm 51 and make that your model prayer. It was what King David prayed when he called on God's mercy after his sins were exposed.

It is my sincere hope that you have made peace with God—that you have dealt with what God sees as your life-threatening problem. Now, we will look at your splinter.

The Advantages of Panic Attacks

I was once speaking to about thirty people about their salvation. Most didn't want to hear what I was saying. I knew that, because my son-in-law and I had been preaching at the local courthouse almost every day for two years. Although we were always polite in what we said, we knew that most in line would rather not have us there. They were lined up, waiting to see the judge. What we saw as a God-given opportunity for people to hear the message of everlasting life, they saw as a nuisance.

Sitting directly in front of me as I spoke was a man wearing sunglasses and holding a white cane. He was evidently blind. I remember thinking how he wasn't looking at passing cars or reading literature. He couldn't. He was just sitting there, listening to the claims of the Gospel. His blindness meant that he wasn't distracted by other things. In that sense, the blind man had a great advantage over the sighted people. He was able to listen to the message of everlasting life, without distraction.

Your panic attacks give you a great advantage over people who have never been humbled and brought to their knees by fear. They are proud, confident, and independent, and they therefore don't think that they need

God. They think that they are insightful, and that thought adds to their blindness. But your weakness has made you open your heart to the claims of the Gospel without any distractions.

Imagine if God took a moment to show you what your life would have been without the attacks that plague you. He lifts you into a vision of your success, confidence, and independence, and shows you the end of your life where you ignored His mercy. He shows you dying in your sins and ending up in Hell. Forever.

Then He shows you a vision of where you will end up as a direct result of the panic attacks. They brought you to your knees, and that brought you to the foot of the Cross. Can you see that? If you have made peace with God, then can you thank Him for the attacks? It is the irritation in the oyster that creates the pearl. Thank God for the horrible irritation of irrational fear. Thank Him from your heart.

When someone becomes a Christian, they enter into a very real spiritual realm.

So the question arises, "Are panic attacks spiritual, or are they your mind playing tricks on you?" No one knows for sure the answer to this question. Each case is different. Some attacks may be natural, triggered by natural circumstances. Others may be spiritual, triggered by what the Bible calls a fear that has torment. However, I have found that when I have been in the middle of an attack, I wasn't too concerned about exactly where it was coming from. If I hit my thumb with a hammer, I don't really care what angle the hammer came from. All I really care about is getting rid of the pain. No doubt that's how you feel about the pain an attack brings. So, let's look at how to deal with the pain of an attack. Then we will look at where I think attacks come from.

Getting a Panic Attack Under Control

The moment we have an attack, we tend to unconsciously over-breathe. This is known as hyperventilation. This brings with it accompanying symptoms. They range from light headedness (giddiness), shortness of breath, heart palpitations, numbness, chest pains, dry mouth, clammy hands, difficulty swallowing, shaking, sweating, feeling weak, and tiredness.

During a panic attack, each of these symptoms feeds off the other. The most important thing to understand about hyperventilation is that although it can make us feel that we don't have enough oxygen, the opposite is actually happening. We are getting too much oxygen. The fight or flight reaction (a panic attack) is causing your body to take in too much. We need a certain amount of carbon dioxide, but when we hyperventilate, we don't give our body long enough to retain the carbon dioxide, and it doesn't use the oxygen we have. This causes a feeling of shortness of breath, when we actually have too much. That sets into motion confusion and many of the above symptoms.

So, here are some ways to counteract this:

Breathe in through your nose, and then breathe slowly out through your mouth. If you feel an attack coming on, inhale very deeply through your nose, until you feel as though you are going to burst. As you exhale, slowly release air through your mouth as though you are whistling. Do this five times. That *will* help you. It puts the right amount of oxygen back into your blood and therefore into your brain. This may make you feel a little dizzy, but it will help your thoughts come more clearly.

A panic attack releases adrenalin and increases the heart rate, which pumps blood and oxygen through the brain. This should be happening so that you can flee from danger, but because there is no danger, it brings confusion to the mind and produces more fear.

Hold your breath for ten or fifteen seconds. Repeat a few times. This is another way to bring back the right level of oxygen.

Breathe in and out of a paper bag. This will cause you to re-inhale the carbon dioxide that you exhaled.

Walk briskly or jog while breathing through the nose. This will also counter hyper-ventilation. If you find that your breathing pattern is irregular or uncomfortable, the best way to "reset" it is by exercising. Start off gradually and build on it. Regular exercise will help to decrease general stress levels, and this decreases the chance of panic attacks.

Breathe deeply from your diaphragm. You can also practice a special type of breathing. This is a breathing that goes deep into your diaphragm (the area below your chest). The out breath must be longer that the in breath. This causes stimulation of the part of your nervous system responsible for relaxation. If you breathe in this way then your body will have no choice but to relax·

It may take a few minutes, but the body will respond regardless of what your mind is thinking. Try this now. Sit down and close your eyes. Become aware of your breathing … and breathe in to the count of seven … and breathe out to the count of eleven. You can hold for a couple of seconds at the bottom of the out breath if that's comfortable for you.

It may be a little difficult at first, but doing this regularly will cause your general anxiety level to come down. The relaxation of breathing is perhaps why Yoga is so popular among those who are stressed. It's not the Yoga that's beneficial, but the simple breathing techniques that come with it.

If you practice this technique regularly, you may find that you begin to breathe this way automatically, if you feel anxious. Regular relaxation inhibits the production of stress hormones in the body, so it actually becomes more difficult to slip into a panic. If you practice this daily, hyperventilating should cease to be a problem. This will give you more control over panic attacks.

The Power of Distraction

Agoraphobia (fear of going into the public) can also develop as panic attacks spread from one situation to another. The attack works through the unconscious mind. We unconsciously think that we see a pattern that was previously associated with panic, and we assume that it is appropriate to panic again.

For example, a lady has her first attack on a crowded underground train when it became stuck in a tunnel. Her mother has just died, and she is already highly stressed. The following week she has another attack when she is sitting on a sofa surrounded by people. Her unconscious mind has decided that this is the same situation as the underground (where she had been sitting surrounding by people) and triggers a second occurrence. From then on, she begins to avoid sitting down and being surrounded by people. Her fear spreads.

You may have experienced something similar. You may have had an attack in front of someone, and that left you feeling humiliated. You had no explanation for the person who saw you paralyzed by fear. You try to forget that horrible experience. You never want it to happen to you again.

Some time later you are at a store, not thinking about anything but what you have to purchase. Suddenly you see a friend approaching you, and you hear, "How are you doing?" Immediately you think, "Oh no! I hope I don't have a panic attack right now and humiliate myself again." That simple thought can be enough to trigger an attack. If that happens, the next time you are in public the thought that someone is going to come up to you and trigger another attack becomes ever stronger. The fear consumes and paralyzes you. So, you decide to deal with the problem by staying at home.

One answer to this dilemma is to go into the public arena, but to carry something special in your pocket, wallet or in your purse. It doesn't matter what it is, a picture, a booklet—something you have in your hand that is "remarkable." It is something that you can *remark* about. It may be from the store

... *anything* that will get the attention off you, and onto the object. You simply greet the person and say, "How are you doing? Did you see this?" You show the booklet, picture, or object to your friend, and then you say, "Well, it was nice to see you. I must get going. I'll see you later."

Just making that small provision of having an object that will take the attention off you will help you immensely. This is because it is a way of escape for you. You have the knowledge that there is a way out of a panic attack if you meet someone. It really does work, because it will help to put you back into the control seat.

Scaling Panic Attacks Down

Something else that may help you is to make a habit of scaling your attack. A full blown attack is a "Ten." A mild attack is a "One." By scaling anxiety in this way, you are putting a fence around the experience so that the limits are clear. This will help to separate yourself further from the experience. It will put you *outside* of the attack—more like an observer. This will help to give you more of a sense of control. You could carry a pen and paper to scale it. You will have to be resolute about doing this because you may not be able to think clearly when you have an attack. As you well know, the fear is totally irrational. It comes from left field. It's not the *rational* part of the brain that deals with panic attacks. This is why people often find it hard to make decisions during an attack. So, make your mind up that you are going to get your pen and paper out, and decide that you are going to stay calm. Then go with the experience, so that (as an observer), you can scale it. Fighting it, becoming angry or becoming more fearful will just fuel the fire. This attitude of being an observer tells the mind that you are not really threatened. You are in control.

Louisa May Alcott said, "I'm not afraid of storms, for I'm learning how to sail my ship."

I Don't Do Counseling

You may have heard that becoming a Christian is a way to overcome life's problems. Preachers talk of success, of health, real happiness, and overcoming life's problems, etc. They tell us that God is the answer to every human dilemma. In one sense, it's true. As a Christian, I can cast all my care upon God. He will give me peace in the storm. I can trust Him at the Red Sea or in a lion's den. But to say that Christians don't have the same problems as everyone else, just isn't true. I know because my panic attacks started when I was a Christian. Let me give you the details.

Rarely do I become involved in counseling; I leave that to the expertise of the local pastor. However, I was awakened one morning by my wife, Sue. She said, "There is someone in

21

the living room and he desperately wants to talk to you." I protested, "But it's not even seven A.M. ... and I don't do counseling!"

Nevertheless, I made my way into the living room and found a man whose eyes flashed with despair. I had met him a few months earlier when he purchased a series of our tapes, but this day he looked like a different man. It turned out that his whole life seemed to be falling to pieces. There were terrible problems at work, at home, and even in his church. Everything had suddenly gone wrong. I looked him in the eye and asked, "You didn't pray that God would 'break' you, did you?"[1] He looked back at me and said, "I asked God to break me and grind me to powder ..."

The Refining Fire
Make sure you realize what you are saying at church when you sing words from songs like a Christian song that was popular in the 1980s and 90s: "Refiner's fire, my heart's one desire is to be holy." I used to hum the song. Let me tell you why. We may think that we are asking God for the "warm fuzzies," but the *refining fire* is what Job[2] went through,

and God may just give you your heart's one desire if you keep asking Him. After the church service, you find that someone has just crashed into your new car. That week you discover that God has let the devil get at you and your house has burned to the ground, your spouse and children have been killed, and someone forgot to pay the insurance premium.

The loss of your family, car, and home, and financial collapse give you a complete nervous breakdown. Well, rejoice—because you are getting your heart's one desire. Read the Book of Job. I've been through the Refiner's fire, and I never want to go through it again. My prayer is, "If it is possible, let this cup pass from me." Jesus had to suffer; there was no alternative for Him. But there is an alternative for us. If we chasten ourselves, perhaps God will not chasten us. Instead of praying that God will break me, I say, "Please, Lord, be gentle on your servant. 'Neither chasten me in your hot displeasure' [Psalm 38.11]. Help me to see areas that I need to change."

If we discipline ourselves to pray and read and obey God's Word, we may avoid the Refiner's fire. If we draw close to Him, we won't need a lion's den to bring us to our knees. If we scatter abroad, preaching the Word everywhere, we may not need a Saul of Tarsus to breathe out slaughter against us.[3] If we cut off unfruitful branches, we won't feel the pain of the Husbandman's sharp pruning sheers. Read the last chapters of Job and learn the lesson, so that you won't have to go through the earlier chapters. Scripture was written for our instruction. Lay your hand on your mouth and quickly bow to the sovereignty of God.

The Fiery Trial

Let me share something very personal. In June 1985, I had just finished preaching in a small country church when a lean-looking young man approached me and said, "I wish I was like you." I managed a smile, but held onto the words that came to mind. *You don't know what you are saying.* Little did he know that at that moment, I was going through sheer terror. I had been in a back room praying earlier that day, when suddenly it seemed that all Hell was let loose in my mind. It was as though God had removed every hedge of protection from me and a thousand demons of terror invaded my thoughts. I fell upon the floor. I wept. I cried out to God. I exorcised myself, to no avail. It was like a living nightmare. There is no way I can describe the experience of the following months, other than to say that it was like being held over a black pit of insanity by a spider's web.

When I arrived home from that series of meetings, my wife, Sue, asked how they went. I said, "The meetings were fine." Then I broke down in tears. I felt so crushed within my mind that I was unable to have family devotions (something our family had had for years). I couldn't even eat a meal at the table with my family for over twelve months. The experience of sitting opposite someone was too traumatic. The thought of it terrified me.

As a mature Christian, I was able to diagnose myself. I had a "wounded spirit." I had prayed for years that God would use me to reach out to the lost, and before He could use me, I needed to have a broken spirit:

> *But this is the man to whom I will look and have regard: he who is humble and of a broken or wounded spirit, and who trembles at My word and reveres My commands (Isaiah 66:2, Amplified Bible).*

It was A.W. Tozer who said, "Before God uses a man, God will break the man." It took years to overcome that experience. At one point, I couldn't even gather enough courage to go to my home church. I wanted to, but irrational fear was paralyzing me. The first Sunday after the initial experience, I was in my bedroom trying to gather the courage to go with my family to church. The fear was so strong, I would actually lose my breath from it even while I lay in bed. As I lay there, my seven-year-old son came into the bedroom and handed me a note. He had written out a few Scriptures he thought I should read, although he had no idea what I was going through. These were the verses:

> *The Lord is my helper, and I will not fear what man shall do to me (Hebrews 13:6).*

*But the path of the just is as the shining
light that shines more and more unto
the perfect day (Proverbs 4:18).*

*Greater is he that is in you, than he
that is in the world (1 John 4:4).*

Then he had written the words, "I love
you, Dad!"

I can't tell you how consoling those
verses were to me. I thought that I was losing
my mind. Just to know that God had any
concern for what I was going though was a
great comfort. Read them and make them
your own. Let them comfort you also. If you
are trusting in the Savior, you are not alone.
Those promises are yours.

How to Speed Up the Process

Perhaps you know the Lord, and there has been a cry in your heart to be used by God. How can you do nothing when the world is going to Hell? You know that you must warn them. Now you find yourself in a dark and frightening part of your life. However, if you understand why it is happening and what you can do to speed up the process, it will certainly be a great help.

If God in His great wisdom sees fit to use the Refiner's fire (if He takes you through a fiery trial), then it is only "if need be" (see 1 Peter 1:6). Pray that you may avoid it, but this is often normal procedure in being prepared to be used by the Lord. A wild horse is no good to a rider. It can't be trusted. It needs its spirit broken so that it will willingly yield to the desire of the rider. So, let me share with you a few words of comfort so that if you are finding that you are hanging over a dark chasm of insanity by the spider web of faith, you will know why, and you will realize that the web is unbreakable.

Those who are unsaved and experience panic attacks are often driven to drugs, alcohol, hopeless despair, or insanity. Many no doubt commit suicide. The Christian who suffers doesn't do so in vain. The Bible makes that clear. But there is a sense of guilt on top of the fear. The experience doesn't seem to match the Bible's description of a faith-filled Christian. He says, "I *will not* fear"... *and yet he still fears*. His will is incapacitated.

If you are having anxiety attacks and you have prayed, and prayed, and prayed for deliverance, and still find yourself in such a predicament, there are strong consolations.

Comfort for the Christian

The apostle Paul was no stranger to fear. He said, "For, when we were come to Macedonia, our flesh had no rest, but we were troubled on every side; without were fightings, *within were fears*" (2 Corinthians 7:5, emphasis added).

Look at these verses from 2 Corinthians 12:7-9:

> *And lest I should be exalted above measure through the abundance of the revelations, there was given to me a thorn in the flesh, the messenger of Satan to buffet me, lest I should be exalted above measure. For this thing I besought the Lord thrice, that it might depart from me. And he said to me, My grace is sufficient for you: for my strength is made perfect in weakness. Most gladly therefore will I rather glory in my infirmities, that the power of Christ may rest upon me.*

Paul asked for deliverance from this demonic attack three times. Yet, God chose to leave him with it. Some say his thorn in the flesh was a sickness, but that doesn't seem to be what the Bible teaches. It says it was a "messenger of Satan" (a demon) that buffeted him.

Why then did God allow demonic oppression to come against His apostle? He wanted to use Paul, but He didn't want him to fall through pride and fail in his calling. The demonic oppression was to keep him humble as God gave him an abundance of revelations. He had to remain small in his own eyes. The Greek word for "buffet" is *kolaphizo*, which means to *"rap with the fist."* Its root word is *kolos*, which means, "dwarf."

Satan fires arrows only at those who have potential for the Kingdom of God. You have great potential to be used by God in these days. Instead of saying, "But God can't use me when I am paralyzed by fear," say, "Because His strength is made perfect in my weakness, God can use me for His glory *because the fear I am plagued by actually keeps me in weakness.* My fear *makes* me pray. I can't do anything without Him."

Examining Yourself
The Bible says that God will cause everything that happens to the Christian to work together for his or her good, if we are called according

to His purposes (see Romans 8:28). Today, there are many who name the name of Christ, but who never "depart from iniquity." They are not called according to His purposes. They are false converts who "ask Jesus into their heart," but are actually unconverted because they have never truly repented. So, it is important that you examine yourself to see if you are in the faith (see 2 Corinthians 13:5). Those who allow sin in their lives are actually opening themselves up to demonic influence. The Bible instructs us to "neither give place to the devil" (Ephesians 4:27).

Again, afflictions only work together for our good, if we are "called according to [God's] purpose." Are we, as professing Christians, doing that which is pleasing to God? Therefore, the following are questions each of us needs to ask ourselves:

Do I honor my parents? Do I value them implicitly? God commands that we honor our parents, and then the Scriptures warn, "that it may be well with you, and you may live long on the earth" (Ephesians 6:3). In other words, if you don't value your parents, all will not be well with you. I have found that many people have demonic problems because they hate their parents.

Is there any unconfessed sin in my life? Is there any bitterness, resentment, or jealousy? Has someone hurt me in the past whom I can't find it within my heart to forgive? Then I am giving place to the devil. If I won't forgive and forget, I'm like a man who is stung to death by one bee. You could understand someone being stung to death by a *swarm* of bees, but we can do something about one bee. The sad thing about someone who becomes bitter is that all they need to do to deal with their problem is to swat the thing through repentance. God says He will not forgive us if we will not forgive from our heart (see Matthew 6:15).

Has there been any occult activity in my life in the past? Do I have idols (even as souvenirs) in my home? Go through your home and get rid of anything that you don't have peace about.

Is there any pornography in my life? I need to prayerfully walk around in the house and ask God if there is *anything* that is unpleasing to Him. Then I must consider the same thing within the temple of my own body.

Am I a glutton? Do I feed filth into my mind through my eyes or through my ears? Do my hands touch only what is pleasing in His sight? Are my words kind and loving? Are the meditations of my mind pleasing to God?

The only way to know if you are genuine in your Christian walk is by examining "fruit." There are a number of fruits in Scripture: the fruit of praise, the fruit of thanksgiving, the fruit of holiness, the fruit of repentance, the fruit of righteousness, and the fruit of the Spirit—love, joy, peace, patience, goodness, gentleness, faith, meekness, and temperance. Are these evident in my life?

The Theory of Relativity
A key to overcoming trials is to understand that they are relative. The next time you feel sorry for yourself after an attack, ask yourself, "Would I like to trade places with someone who has an agonizing terminal disease? Would I like to trade places with a burn victim who has been burned over

90 percent of his body?" We can't imagine the agonies those in such predicaments go through. Have you ever burned yourself on a toaster? Think what it might be like for those poor people. Such sober thoughts bring our problems into perspective, and should make us want to thank God for His many blessings. Not only for what we have, but also for those things we don't have—like unspeakable bodily pain.

The fruit of thanksgiving should be evident in the Christian, not only for temporal blessings, but also for the Cross. Paul was persecuted beyond measure. He was whipped 39 times for his faith, on five separate occasions (see 2 Corinthians 11:24), yet he said "Thanks be to God for his unspeakable gift" (2 Corinthians 9:13). He didn't complain. He thanked God for his salvation. He knew that God would work everything out for his good.

As Christians, we should have the fruit of holiness. We should be separated from this evil world, to God. We should have evidence of our repentance. If we have stolen, we will return what isn't ours. We will set right (where possible) that which we have wronged. Lastly, we will possess the fruit of the Spirit. If we are rooted and grounded in Him, we will have the fruits of His character hanging from the branches of our lives. Do we have love that cares for others? Do we care enough about the salvation of sinners to put feet to our prayers and take the Gospel to them? Love is not passive. It will not be self-indulgent while others suffer. It is empathetic. Are you sure that you are saved? Many won't bother to examine themselves to make their calling and election sure. They will wait until the Day of Judgment. That may be too late.

The Light Affliction

Perhaps you have carefully examined yourself, and you have concluded that you *are* in the faith. You have made a clean cut with sin and with this world. So, what then is the devil doing in our lives if we haven't given "place" to him? There must be good reason for him to be there. The only reasonable conclusion is that God has given permission. This happened in the book of Job.[4] God allowed Satan to buffet Job so that he would grow in his faith in God. As I have said before, the Bible says that the Book of Job is for our admonition and instruction.

Study the following verse from the *Amplified Bible*:

It is God who is all the while effectually at work in you [energizing

> *and creating in you the power and*
> *desire], both to will and to work for*
> *His good pleasure and satisfaction*
> *and delight (Philippians 2:13).*

We have established that God is at work in you. You have this demonic "buffeting" from which God will not presently deliver you, because He is doing a good work in you. Therefore, what should be your attitude to this good work He is doing? It should be one of joy—*because your joy is evidence of how much you trust God*. If you trust Him, then you will rejoice for His goodness, and that joy will be strength to you.

Take for instance a world champion boxer. His coach loves him to a point where he wants him above all things to be a winner. So, what does the coach do—buy him a sofa, a TV, and potato chips? No. Instead, he places weights on his shoulders and resistance against his arms. He will even look around for the toughest sparring partner he can find. If the boxer doesn't understand what his trainer is doing, if he doesn't have faith in his methods, he will get depressed and lose heart. But if he knows what's going on, he will rejoice now in the trials because he sees, through the eyes of faith, the finished product.

That's why God is letting the devil loose on you. It's to make you strong. Paul says,

> *For our light affliction, which is but for a moment [in the light of eternity], works for us a far more exceeding and eternal weight of glory (2 Corinthians 4:17).*

Afflictions work *for* us, not against us, if we are in God's will. How is your joy when the Trainer brings the resistance your way? How is your attitude to God just after a panic attack? How much faith do you have in Him? The joy you have will be your measuring rod.

Spurgeon on Despair and Fear
I was encouraged to read where my favorite preacher (C. H. Spurgeon) also went through a deep pit of despair. Here is his experience:[5]

> *Believer, if the conversion of the world rested with the Church, if the*

*out gathering of the elect depended
upon us, it never would be done; but
God makes us work for this end, and
so He works first in us, and then He
works with us. How this ought to
encourage us to work!*

*This little arm, what can it do? But
that eternal arm, what can it not do?
This tongue, how feebly can it speak;
but the voice of Him who spoke as
never man spoke, how persuasively
can it speak? Our spirits, narrow and
limited, what can they affect? But
His unbounded Spirit, what cannot
He perform?*

*Oh! let everyone here who has been
serving his Master bid farewell to
everything like a discouraging or
desponding thought. The great army
of God is not defeated; it never can
be, in the long run it must conquer.
And even those parts of the divine
strategy of our great Commander
which looked like retreat, are only
portions of His perpetual victory. He*

*is fighting on, and will win the battle,
even to the end.*

*It is a great consolation to the believer
to know that Jesus lives, and lives in
triumph. I do remember, and I cannot
help repeating what I have told you
before—I do remember, when in
an hour of the most overwhelming
sorrow through which a mind could
pass, this one thing restored and
comforted me. After that dreadful
catastrophe in the Surrey Gardens,
my mind gave way and my sorrow
was extreme—I had almost lost my
reason for some three weeks, and was
desponding and brokenhearted. I was
alone, walking in solitude, mourning,
and weeping as I did day and night,
and all of a sudden there came
into my mind, as though it dropped
from Heaven, this text: "Him hath
God highly exalted and given him
a name which is above every name
that at the name of Jesus every knee
should bow." You know the rest. The
thought that crossed my mind was
this: I am one of his soldiers, and*

I am lying in a ditch to die. It does not matter; the King has won the victory—Christ has won the victory—Christ is to the fore. If I die like a dog, I care not. The crown is on His head. He is safely exalted.

In a moment, I was happy; my trouble was gone; I found myself perfectly restored; I fell on my knees in a solitary place, praising God who, in infinite mercy, had made that text to be a balm to my spirit. Now there may be someone here who feels much as I did—disconsolate, cast down. If you really love Jesus, there is not a nobler balm for your care than this: He reigns, He is glorious; the government is not taken from His shoulders. Our King is no captive; our Emperor has not yielded up his sword: our Prince Imperial is not banished: our Empire never fails, the city of Jerusalem is not besieged: there shall be no straightness of bread in her streets. "God is in the midst of her: she shall not be moved; God shall help her, and that right early."

Let the heathen rage: let the people and nations be moved: let the whole earth rock and reel, and the mountains be carried into the midst of the sea, God is our refuge and strength, our very present help in time of trouble. God reigns, and the kingdom of Jesus is settled by an unchangeable decree. Therefore lift up your heads, you saints, for your redemption draws near, and even now clap your joyful hands, and go back again to the conflict of life until your Master calls you home like true heroes, that henceforth shall know no fear, and shall never turn your backs in the day of battle. God grant it may be so for His name's sake. Amen.[6]

Can you see what Spurgeon is saying? He is saying to get your mind off yourself. To do that you need to have faith in God and in His promises. If you lack the sort of faith that can lift you out of the pit, and set your feet on the mountain of thanksgiving, I will share something a little later that will help you. In the meanwhile, here is some more insight as to where trials often come from:

For you, Oh God, have proved us:
you have tried us, as silver is tried.
You have caused men to ride over
our heads, we went through fire
and through water: but you brought
us out into a wealthy place (Psalm
66:10,12).

God takes us through the fires of
persecution, tribulation, and temptation to
purify us, not to burn us. He takes us through
water to cleanse us, not to drown us. Look at
the reason God chastens His children, given
in Hebrews 12:9-15:

Furthermore, we have had fathers
of our flesh, which corrected us, and
we gave them reverence: shall we
not much rather be in subjection to
the Father of spirits, and live? For
they verily for a few days chastened
us after their own pleasure; but he
for our profit, that we might be
partakers of his holiness. Now no
chastening for the present seems to
be joyous, but grievous: nevertheless,
afterward it yields the peaceable fruit
of righteousness to them, which are

exercised thereby. Wherefore lift up the hands, which hang down, and the feeble knees; and make straight paths for your feet, lest that which is lame be turned out of the way; but let it rather be healed. Follow peace with all men, and holiness, without which no man shall see the Lord: looking diligently lest any man fail of the grace of God; lest any root of bitterness springing up trouble you, and thereby many be defiled.

Getting Yourself Together

In other words, get it together. Don't fall into discouragement, which is essentially a lack of faith in God. *Dis*-couragment is your courage taken from you. Don't let that happen to you. *Keep* the faith. If you let your arms hang down in depression instead of rejoicing that God is working all things out for your good, you are saying that God isn't faithful, that His promises aren't worth believing, that He is actually a liar. There is no greater insult to God than to not believe His promises. The result of unbelief will be depression, discouragement, self-pity, and resentment, then bitterness, which you will end up spreading to others.

If you have never thanked God for His promises, for His faithfulness, for the fact that He is working with you, in you, and for you—if you have been joyless, or even despised what has been happening to you and moved into bitterness—then repent of the sin of mistrust. How insulted you would be if you were a faithful and loving trainer, and your boxer, for whose good you are laboring, began to despise you for what you were doing.

On the other hand, if you are "exercised thereby," the result will be the "peaceable fruit of righteousness." In other words, you will end up living a life that is in complete righteousness, and bring a smile to the heart of your heavenly Father.

Look at Hebrews 12:11 (in the verses we have just read). Notice the word "afterward." That one word was my light in the dark tunnel. It meant there was an end to my terror. It meant that the light at the end of the tunnel that wasn't another train heading for me. Write down the word "afterward," and put it somewhere where you will be reminded that you have hope—and "hope never disappoints or deludes or shames us" (Romans 5:5, *Amplified*).

Guard yourself against condemnation.

When I was paralyzed through fear, I could hear myself saying, "What's wrong with you! Pull yourself together. Have faith in God." But I still had panic attacks. I had to remind myself that I was no less spiritual than those who seemed to have complete victory over their fears. If you don't believe it, think of the experience of Oswald Chambers, author of the mega-bestselling devotional, *My Utmost For His Highest*. Now there's a man whose life and words have been an inspiration to millions. He was "spiritual" in the truest sense of the word. However, the great author had four years in his life of which he said,

> *"God used me during those years for the conversion of souls, but I had no conscious communion with Him. The Bible was the dullest, most uninteresting book in existence."*[7]

Look at his words. He was in such despair that even the promises of God didn't encourage him. He described those four years as "hell on earth." However, he found that there was an "afterward," saying,

> *But those of you who know the experience know very well how God brings one to the point of utter despair, and I got to the place where I did not care whether everyone knew how bad I was, I cared not for another on earth, saving to get out of my present condition.*[8]

If you have panic attacks or agoraphobia (the fear of being in public), don't fall into the deep pit of self-pity, because it has ugly bedfellows—discouragement, joylessness, condemnation, despair, and hopelessness. The sides of the pit of self-pity are very slippery, but there is one firm foothold. It is the uplifting staircase of something on which we have briefly touched. In the next chapter, we will look at how you can get your foot into it.

Pinch the Nose

ue and I were visiting an elderly lady named Helen, a 93-year-old who had broken her hip. She was unhappy because the food in the convalescent home wasn't very good. One day Mary walked into Helen's room. Mary was in her late seventies and had to be permanently fed through a tube that ran from a bottle directly into her stomach. Mary never tasted food or drink, and barring a miracle from God, she would never taste food or liquid again. Mary's condition made Helen thankful that at least she could have the pleasure of food and drink, even if it wasn't up to standard.

Then there was Robert. Robert could eat any food he wanted. He had a good clear brain, but he had chronic emphysema. He couldn't breathe. Whenever I looked into his room, he was sitting on his bed, leaning over with his hand on his forehead. He gasped for every breath twenty-four hours a day. Robert's problem made Mary thankful that at least she could breathe.

You and I need to be continually reminded that we don't have to look too far for people who are suffering so badly that their problems dwarf ours. If you don't believe me, try being Robert for two minutes. Pinch your nose with one hand. Then, with the other one, hold your lips together so that a meager amount of air gets into your mouth. Don't cheat. Do that for 120 long seconds. Feel the sweat break out on your forehead. Feel the panic. After two minutes of gasping for breath, when you let go, you will begin to thank God that you can breathe, that you can eat. That will bring your problems into perspective. I'm not demeaning your fears. I'm offering you a way to lift yourself out of the pit of self-pity.

So next time you are attacked in some way, pull yourself together with a prayer of heartfelt thanksgiving, and say:

Father, I thank You that all things work together for my good; that it is You who are at work in me to will and do of Your good pleasure. Your strength is made perfect in my weakness. I will not let this attack discourage me, because Your grace is sufficient for me. You will help me through it. When I think of the sufferings of many, many others, I feel ashamed for having any self-pity. I will therefore rejoice in the God of my salvation and give You sincere thanks in and for everything. In Jesus' name, I pray. Amen.

Your Deep Roots

Your constant battle with trials will make you no stranger to them. Like a tree that is continuously beaten about by the wind, your roots will be deep. You will find, if you have an acquaintance with fear, etc., that you can live with it when others can't. You will be able to do things that others can't. The roots of your faith in God will be deeper than the roots of those who have never been ravaged by the winds of terror. Again, affliction works *for* us. God doesn't let the wind blow to destroy, but to strengthen. You will be able to go places and do things that others would fear to do, because those things that should (rationally) produce fear pale in significance compared to the average attack of irrational fear.

Again, do you believe God is at work in you to will and do of His good pleasure? Then rejoice, and let the joy of the Lord be your strength. There is a world weighed in the balance and found wanting. Don't fiddle while Rome burns. Your problems and fears are nothing compared to the terrible plight of the sinner. Eternal Hell is his destiny. Lift up hands that hang down, lift up your heart through faith, then lift up your voice like a trumpet and show this people their transgressions.

The Inner Ear Imbalance

I received the following letter from someone who had suffered from panic attacks, but had been helped in another way:

> *I was looking over one of my mother's books,* The Way of the Master, *and read your preface: "One year later, I entered into the deepest, darkest,*

most frightening time of my life as I began to suffer ongoing episodes of irrational fear. These panic attacks left me so broken that for more than a year, I couldn't even eat a meal with my family. It took five long years to recover from those experiences."

I have suffered from these, too. My journey to discovering what causes panic attacks and how they can be treated was painful, but might be invaluable to others who suffer from them.

The information I discovered during the "most frightening time of my life" also came from a book about home health remedies. I looked up panic attacks (it took me four months of research and misdiagnoses from doctors before I could even place a name on what was wrong with me: Panic Disorder) in the index and ran across a blurb in that section that claimed ninety percent of all panic attacks were caused by inner ear disturbance. The doctor making this claim is Dr. Harold Levinson. His

*office is in Great Neck, New York.
He wrote a book called* Phobia Free.
*It's available on Amazon for about
three bucks, used. It should also
be available at any larger library.
The very first medication listed in
that book is Meclezine (Antivert). I
tricked my doctor into prescribing
it to me, and within 45 minutes
of taking the first dose, I felt like
someone had lifted a thousand pound
weight off my shoulders. Turns out I
could have obtained Meclezine OTC
(over the counter) by simply asking
for it at the drugstore. It costs about
six bucks a hundred.*

*Dr. Harold Levinson and his book
saved my physical life. The fate of
my immortal soul is yet another
topic. Ray, your brief description of
your symptoms indicates possible
agoraphobia. Even though the book
title is* Phobia Free, *there are many
case histories in there that contain
panic attacks.*

Sincerely, Paul H.

Review

So let's stop for a minute, and summarize what we have looked at in this book.

1. Get perspective. Panic attacks are no problem compared to our bigger problem— our relationship to God. A splinter in the thumb is nothing compared to a severed jugular vein. I trust that you have dealt with that problem.

2. Control your intake of oxygen through controlled breathing.

3. The power of distraction. When you go into public, take something with you that will take the attention off yourself.

4. Exercise.

5. Carry a pen and paper, and scale your attacks. This will make you an "observer" and give you more control.

6. Sincerely thank God that He's working in you to do His will.

7. Bring your problems into perspective by remembering Robert (who *suffered* from emphysema), and thanking God for what you *haven't* got.

More Food

gain, I hope and pray that you haven't come this far without making peace with God. There is nothing more important. This chapter and the ones following are additional principles that can help you grow as a Christian.[9]

A healthy baby has a healthy appetite. If you have truly been "born" of the Spirit of God, you will have a healthy appetite. We are told, "As newborn babes, desire the pure milk of the Word, that you may grow thereby" (1 Peter 2:2). Feed yourself daily without fail. Job said, "I have treasured the words of His mouth more than my necessary food" (Job 23:12). The more you eat, the quicker you will grow, and the less bruising you will have. Speed up the process and save yourself some pain—vow to read God's Word

59

every day, without fail. Say to yourself, "No Bible, no breakfast. No read, no feed." Be like Job, and put your Bible *before* your belly. If you do that, God promises that you will be like a fruitful, strong, and healthy tree (see Psalm 1). Each day, find somewhere quiet and thoroughly soak your soul in the Word of God. There may be times when you read through its pages with great enthusiasm, and other times when it seems dry and even boring. But food profits your body whether you enjoy it or not. As a child, you no doubt ate desserts with great enthusiasm. Perhaps vegetables weren't so exciting. If you were a normal child, you probably had to be encouraged to eat them at first. Then, as you matured in life, you learned to discipline yourself to eat vegetables. This is because they physically benefit you, even though they may not bring pleasure to your taste buds.

Faith—Elevators Can Let You Down

When a young man once said to me, "I find it hard to believe some of the things in the Bible," I smiled and asked, "What's your name?" When he said, "Paul," I casually answered, "I don't believe you." He looked at me questioningly. I repeated, "What's your name?" Again he said, "Paul," and again I answered, "I don't believe you." Then I asked, "Where do you live?" When he told me, I said, "I don't believe that either." His reaction, understandably, was anger. I said, "You look a little upset. Do you know why? You're upset because I didn't believe what you told me. If you tell me that your name is Paul, and I say, 'I don't believe you,' it means that I think you are a liar. You are trying to deceive me by telling me your name is Paul, when it's not."

Then I asked him if he, a mere man, felt insulted by my lack of faith in his word, how much more does he insult Almighty God by refusing to believe His Word? In doing so, he was saying that God isn't worth trusting—that He is a liar and a deceiver. The Bible says, "He who does not believe God has made Him a liar" (1 John 5:10). It also says, "Beware, brethren, lest there be in any of you an evil heart of unbelief ..." (Hebrews 3:12). Martin Luther asked, "What greater insult ... can there be to God, than not to believe His promises?"

I have heard people say, "But I just find it hard to have faith in God," not realizing the implications of their words. These are the same people who often accept the daily weather forecast, believe the newspapers, and trust their lives to pilots they have never seen whenever they board planes. We exercise faith every day. We rely on our car's brakes. We trust history books, medical books, and elevators. Yet, elevators can let us down. History books can be wrong. Planes can crash. How much more then should we trust the sure and true promises of Almighty God. He will never let us down ... if we trust Him.

Cynics often argue, "You can't trust the Bible—it's full of mistakes." It is. The first mistake was when man rejected God, and the Scriptures show men and women making the same tragic mistake again and again.

It's also full of what *seem* to be contradictions. For example, the Scriptures tell us that "with God, nothing shall be impossible" (Luke 1:37); there is nothing Almighty God can't do. Yet we are also told that it is "impossible for God to lie"

(Hebrews 6:18). So there *is* something God cannot do! Isn't that an obvious "mistake" in the Bible?

The answer to this dilemma is found in the lowly worm. Do you know that it would be impossible for me to eat worms? I once saw a man on TV butter his toast, then pour on a can of live, fat, wriggling, blood-filled worms. He carefully took a knife and fork, cut into his moving meal, and ate it. It made me feel sick. It was disgusting. The thought of chewing cold, live worms is so repulsive, so distasteful, I can candidly say it would be impossible for me to eat them, although I have seen it done. It is so abhorrent, I draw on the strength of the word "impossible" to substantiate my claim.

Lying, deception, bearing false witness, etc., is so repulsive to God, so disgusting to Him, so against His holy character, that the Scriptures draw on the strength of the word "impossible" to substantiate the claim. He cannot, could not, and would not lie. That means in a world where we are continually let down, we can totally rely on, trust in, and count on His promises. They are sure, certain, indisputable, true, trustworthy, reliable, faithful, unfailing, dependable, steadfast, and an anchor for the soul. In other words, you can truly believe them, and because of that, you can throw yourself blindfolded and without reserve into His mighty hands. He will never, *ever* let you down. Do you believe that?

Evangelism—Our Most Sobering Task
Late in December 1996, a large family gathered in Los Angeles for a joyous Christmas. There were so many gathered that night, five of the children slept in the converted garage, kept warm during the night by an electric heater placed near the door. During the early hours of the morning, the heater suddenly burst into flames, blocking the doorway. In seconds, the room became a blazing inferno. A frantic 911 call revealed the unspeakable terror as one of the children could be heard screaming, "I'm on fire!" The distraught father rushed into the flames to try to save his beloved children, receiving burns to 50 percent of his body. Tragically, all five children burned to death. They died because steel bars on the windows had thwarted their escape. There was only one door, and it was blocked by the flames.

Imagine you are back in time, just minutes before the heater burst into flames. You peer through the darkness at the peaceful sight of five sleeping youngsters, knowing that at any moment the room will erupt into an inferno and burn the flesh of horrified children. Can you in good conscience walk away? No! You *must* awaken them, and warn them to run from that death trap! If you don't warn them, you are breaking the law.

The world sleeps peacefully in the darkness of ignorance. There is only one Door by which they may escape death. The steel bars of sin prevent their salvation, and at the same time call for the flames of eternal justice. What a fearful thing Judgment Day will be! The fires of the wrath of Almighty God will burn for eternity. The Church has been entrusted with the task of awakening them before it's too late. We cannot turn our backs and walk away in complacency.

Think of how the father ran into the flames. His love knew no bounds. Our devotion to the sober task God has given us will be in direct proportion to our love for the lost. There are only a few who run headlong into the flames to warn them to flee (Luke 10:2).

Please be one of them. We really have no choice. The apostle Paul said, "Woe is me if I do not preach the gospel!" (1 Corinthians 9:16). If you and I ignore a drowning child and let him die when we have the ability to save him, we are guilty of the crime of "depraved indifference." God forbid that any Christian should be guilty of that crime when it comes to those around us who are perishing. We have an obligation to reach out to them. The "Prince of Preachers," Charles Spurgeon, said, "Have you no wish for others to be saved? Then you are not saved yourself. Be sure of that."

A Christian *cannot* be apathetic about the salvation of the world. The love of God in him will motivate him to seek and save that which is lost. You probably have a limited amount of time after your conversion to impact your unsaved friends and family with the Gospel. After the initial shock of your conversion, they will put you in a neat little ribbon-tied box and keep you at arm's length.

So it's important that you take advantage of the short time you have while you still have their ears.

Here's some advice that may save you a great deal of grief. As a new Christian, I did almost irreparable damage by acting like a wild bull in a crystal showroom. I bullied my mom, my dad, and many of my friends into making a "decision for Christ." I was sincere, zealous, loving, kind, and stupid. I didn't understand that salvation doesn't come through making a "decision," but through repentance, and that repentance is God-given (2 Timothy 2:25). The Bible teaches that no one can come to the Son unless the Father "draws" him (John 6:44). If you are able to get a "decision," but the person has no conviction of sin, you will almost certainly end up with a stillborn on your hands. In my "zeal without knowledge," I actually inoculated the very ones I was so desperately trying to reach.

There is nothing more important to you than the salvation of your loved ones, and you don't want to blow it. If you do, you may find that you don't have a second chance. Fervently pray for them, asking God for their salvation. Let them see your faith. Let them feel your kindness, your genuine love, and your gentleness. Buy gifts for no reason. Do chores when you are not asked to. Go the extra mile. Put yourself in their position. You know that you have found everlasting life—*death has lost its sting!* Your joy is unspeakable. But as far as they are concerned, you've been brainwashed and have become part of a weird sect. So your loving actions will speak more loudly than ten thousand eloquent sermons. For this reason you should avoid *verbal* confrontation until you have knowledge that will guide your zeal.

Pray for wisdom and for sensitivity to God's timing. You may have only one shot, so make it count. Keep your cool. If you don't, you may end up with a lifetime of regret. *Believe* me. It is better to hear a loved one or a close friend say, "Tell me about your faith in Jesus Christ," rather than you saying, "Sit down. I want to talk to you." Continue to persevere in prayer for them, that God would open their eyes to the truth.

Remember also that you have the sobering responsibility of speaking to other people's loved ones. Perhaps another Christian has prayed earnestly that God would use a faithful witness to speak to his beloved mom or dad, and *you* are that answer to prayer. You are the true and faithful witness God wants to use. We should share our faith with others *whenever* we can. The Bible says that there are only two times we should do this: "in season and out of season" (2 Timothy 4:2). The apostle Paul pleaded for prayer for his own personal witness. He said,

> *"[Pray] for me, that utterance may be given to me, that I may open my mouth boldly to make known the mystery of the gospel, for which I am an ambassador in chains; that in it I may speak boldly, as I ought to speak" (Ephesians 6:19, 20).*

Never lose sight of the world and all its pains. Keep the fate of the ungodly before your eyes. Too many of us settle down on a padded pew and become introverted. Our world becomes a monastery without walls. Our friends are confined solely to those within the Church, when Jesus was the "friend of sinners." So, take the time to deliberately befriend the lost for the sake of their salvation. Remember that each and every person who dies in his sins has an appointment with the Judge of the Universe. Hell opens wide its terrible jaws. There is no more sobering task than to be entrusted with the gospel of salvation—working with God for the eternal wellbeing of dying humanity.

The Key

Many Christians have thought, *There must be a key to reaching the lost.* There is—and it's rusty through lack of use. The Bible does actually call it "the key," and its purpose is to bring us to Christ, to unlock the Door of the Savior (see John 10:9). Much of the Church still doesn't even know it exists. Not only is it biblical, but it can be shown through history that the Church used it to unlock the doors of revival. The problem is that it was lost around the turn of the twentieth century. Keys have a way of getting lost. Jesus used it. So did Paul (Romans 3:19, 20) and James (James 2:10). Stephen used it when he preached (Acts 7:53). Peter found that it had been used to open the door to release 3,000 imprisoned souls on the Day of Pentecost.

Jesus said that the lawyers had "taken away" the key, and had even refused to use it to let people enter into the Kingdom of God (Luke 11:52). The Pharisees didn't take it away; instead, they bent it out of shape so that it wouldn't do its work (Mark 7:8). Jesus returned it to its true shape, just as the Scriptures prophesied that He would do (Isaiah 42:21).

Satan has tried to prejudice the modern Church against the key. He has maligned it, misused it, twisted it, and, of course, hidden it—he hates it because of what it does. Perhaps you are wondering what this key is. I will tell you. All I ask is that you set aside your traditions and prejudices and look at what God's Word says on the subject.

In Acts 28:23 the Bible tells us that Paul sought to persuade his hearers "concerning Jesus, both out of the law of Moses, and out of the prophets." Here we have two effective means of persuading the unsaved "concerning

Jesus." Let's first look at how the prophets can help persuade sinners concerning Jesus. Fulfilled prophecy *proves* the inspiration of Scripture.

The predictions of the prophets present a powerful case for the inspiration of the Bible. Any skeptic who reads the prophetic words of Isaiah, Ezekiel, Joel, etc., or the words of Jesus in Matthew 24 cannot but be challenged that this is no ordinary book.

The other means by which Paul persuaded sinners concerning Jesus was "out of the law of Moses." We are told that the Law of Moses is good if it is used lawfully (1 Timothy 1:8). It was given by God as a "tutor" to bring us to Christ (Galatians 3:24). Paul wrote that he "would not have known sin except through the law" (Romans 7:7). The Law of God (the Ten Commandments) is evidently the "key of knowledge" Jesus spoke of in Luke 11:52. He was speaking to "lawyers"—those who should have been teaching God's Law so that sinners would receive the "knowledge of sin," and thus recognize their need for the Savior.

Prophecy speaks to the *intellect* of the sinner, while the Law speaks to his *conscience*. One produces *faith* in the Word of God; the other brings *knowledge* of sin in the heart of the sinner. The Law is the God-given "key" to unlock the Door of salvation. You may have noticed that I used this principle in this book.

Prayer—"Wait for a Minute"

As I mentioned earlier in this book, God always answers prayer. Sometimes He says yes; sometimes He says no; and sometimes He says, "Wait for a minute." And since God is outside the dimension of time, a thousand years is the same as a day to Him (see 2 Peter 3:8)—which could mean a ten-year wait for us. So ask in faith, but rest in peace-filled patience.

Surveys show that more than 90 percent of Americans pray daily. No doubt they pray for health, wealth, happiness, etc. They also pray when Grandma gets sick, so when Grandma doesn't get better (or dies), many end up disillusioned or bitter. This is because they don't understand what the Bible says about prayer. It teaches, among other things, that our sin will keep God from even hearing our prayers (Psalm 66:18), and that if we pray with doubt, we will not get an answer (James 1:6,7). Here's how to be heard:

• Pray with faith (Hebrews 11:6).

• Pray with clean hands and a pure heart (Psalm 24:3-4).

• Pray genuine heartfelt prayers, rather than vain repetitions (Matthew 6:7).

• Make sure you are praying to the God revealed in the Scriptures (Exodus 20:3–6).

Praying with Faith

How do you *pray with faith*? If someone says to you, "You have great faith in God," they may think they are paying you a compliment. But they aren't—the compliment is to God. For example, if I said, "I'm a man of great faith in my doctor," it's actually the doctor I'm complimenting. If I have great faith in him, it means that I see him as being a man of integrity, a man of great ability; he is trustworthy. I give "glory" to the man through my faith in him.

The Bible says that Abraham "did not waver at the promise of God through unbelief, but was strengthened in faith, giving glory to God, and being fully convinced that what He had promised He was also able to perform" (Romans 4:20-21). Abraham was a man of great faith in God. Remember, that is not a compliment to Abraham. He merely caught a glimpse of God's incredible ability, His impeccable integrity, and His wonderful faithfulness to keep every promise He makes. Abraham's faith gave "glory" to a faithful God. As far as God is concerned, if you belong to Jesus, you are a VIP. You can boldly come before the throne of grace (Hebrews 4:16). You have access to the King because *you are the son or daughter of the King*. When you were a child, did you have to grovel to get your needs met by your mom or dad? I hope not.

So, when you pray, don't say, "Oh, God, I *hope* you will supply my needs." Instead say something like, "Father, thank You that You keep every promise You make. Your Word says that you will supply *all* my needs according to Your riches in glory by Christ Jesus [Philippians 4:19]. Therefore, I thank

You that You will do this thing for my family. I ask this in the wonderful name of Jesus. Amen."

The great missionary Hudson Taylor said, "Prayer power has never been tried to its full capacity. If we want to see Divine power wrought in the place of weakness, failure, and disappointment, let us answer God's standing challenge, 'Call unto me, and I will answer you, and show you great and mighty things of which you know not of.'"

Clean Hands and a Pure Heart

How do you get *clean hands and a pure heart*? Simply by confessing your sins to God, through Jesus Christ, whose blood cleanses us from all our sin (1 John 1:7–9). When you confess them to God through Jesus, God will not only forgive your every sin, He promises to *forget* them (Hebrews 8:12). He will count it as though you had never sinned in the first place. He will make you pure in His sight—sinless. He will even "purge" your conscience, so that you will no longer have that sense of guilt that you sinned. That's why you need to soak yourself in Holy

Scripture; read the letters to the churches and see the wonderful things God has done for us through the cross of Calvary. If you don't bother to read the "will," you won't have any idea what has been given to you.

Genuine, Heartfelt Prayers

How do you pray *genuine, heartfelt prayers*? Simply by keeping yourself in the love of God. If the love of God is in you, you will never pray hypocritical or selfish prayers. In fact, you won't have to pray selfish prayers if you have a heart of love, because when your prayer life is pleasing to God, He will reward you openly (Matthew 6:6). Just talk to your heavenly Father as candidly and intimately as a young child nestled on Daddy's lap would talk to his earthly father. How would you feel if every day your child pulled out a prewritten statement to dryly recite to you, rather than pouring out the events and emotions of that day? God wants to hear from your heart.

The God of the Scriptures

How do you know you're praying to *the God revealed in Scripture*? Study the Bible.

Don't accept the image of God portrayed by the world, even though it appeals to the natural mind. A loving, kind father figure with no sense of justice or truth appeals to guilty sinners. Look to the thunderings and lightnings of Mount Sinai. Gaze at Jesus on the cross of Calvary—hanging in unspeakable agony because of the justice of a holy God. Such thoughts tend to banish idolatry.

Praise the Lord and Pass the Ammunition

We have been looking at principles for Christian growth. In this chapter, we will look closely at the fact that we are involved in warfare. When you became a Christian, you stepped right into the heat of an age-old battle. You now have a threefold enemy: the world, the devil, and the flesh. Let's look at these three resistant enemies.

The World

Our first enemy is the world. When the Bible speaks of the "world" in this context, it is referring to the sinful, rebellious, world system. This is the world that loves the darkness and hates the light (John 3:20) and is governed by the "prince of the power of the air" (Ephesians 2:2). The Bible says that the Christian has escaped the corruption that is in the world through lust. "Lust" is unlawful desire and is the life blood of the world—whether it be the lust for sexual sin, for power, for money, or for material things. Lust is a monster that will never be gratified, so don't feed it. It will grow bigger and bigger until it weighs heavy upon your back and will be the death of you (James 1:15). There is nothing wrong with sex, power, money, or material things, but when desire for these becomes predominant, it becomes idolatry (Colossians 3:5). We are told, "Do not love the world or the things in the world. If anyone loves the world, the love of the Father is not in him," and, "Whoever therefore wants to be a friend of the world makes himself an enemy of God" (1 John 2:15; James 4:4).

The Devil

The second enemy is the devil. As we have seen, he is known as the "god of this age" (2 Corinthians 4:4). He was your spiritual father before you joined the family of God (John 8:44, Ephesians 2:2). Jesus called the devil a thief who came to steal, kill, and destroy (John 10:10). The way to overcome him and his demons is to make sure you are outfitted with the spiritual armor of God listed in Ephesians 6:10–20. Become intimately familiar with it. Sleep in it. Never take it off. Bind the sword to your hand so you never lose its grip. The reason for this brings us to the third enemy.

The Flesh

The third enemy is what the Bible calls the "flesh." This is your sinful nature. The domain for the battle is your mind. *If you have a mind to*, you *will* be attracted to the world and all its sin. The mind is the control panel for the eyes and the ears, the center of your appetites. All sin begins in the "heart" (Proverbs 4:23; Matthew 15:19). We think of sin before we commit it. The Bible warns that lust brings forth sin, and sin when it's conceived brings forth death. Every day of life, we have a choice. To sin or not to sin—that is the question. The answer to the question of sin is to have the fear of God. If you don't fear God, you will sin to your sinful heart's delight.

Did you know that God kills people? He killed a man for what he did sexually (Genesis 38:9,10), killed another man for being greedy (Luke 12:15–21), and killed a husband and wife for telling one lie (Acts 5:1-10). Knowledge of God's goodness—His righteous judgments against evil—should put the fear of God in us and help us not to indulge in sin. If we know that the eye of the Lord is in every place beholding the evil and the good, and that He will bring every work to judgment, we will live accordingly. Such weighty thoughts are valuable, for "by the fear of the Lord one departs from evil" (Proverbs 16:6). Jesus said,

> *"And I say to you, My friends, do not be afraid of those who kill the body, and after that have no more that they can do. But I will show you whom you should fear: Fear Him who, after He has killed, has power to cast into hell; yes, I say to you, fear Him!" (Luke 12:4, 5)*

Fellowship—Flutter by Butterfly

Pray about where you should fellowship. Make sure the place you select as your church home calls sin what it is—sin. Do they believe the promises of God? Are they loving? Does the pastor treat his wife with respect? Is he a man of the Word? Does he have a humble heart and a gentle spirit? Listen closely to his teaching. It should glorify God, magnify Jesus, and edify the believer. One evidence that you have been truly saved is that you will have a love for other Christians (1 John 3:14). You will want to fellowship with them. The old saying that "birds of a feather flock together" is true of Christians. You gather together for the breaking of bread (communion), for teaching from the Word, and for fellowship. You share the same inspirations, illuminations, inclinations, temptations, aspirations, motivations, and perspirations—you are working together for the same thing: the furtherance of the Kingdom of God on earth. This is why you attend church—not because you have to, but because you want to.

Don't become a "spiritual butterfly." Send your roots down. If you are flitting from church to church, how will your pastor know what type of food you are digesting? We are told that your shepherd is accountable to God for you (Hebrews 13:17), so make yourself known to your pastor. Pray for him regularly. Pray also for his wife, his family, and the church leaders. Being a pastor is no easy task. Most people don't realize how many hours it takes to prepare a fresh sermon each week. They don't appreciate the time spent in prayer and in the study of the Word. If the pastor makes the same joke twice, or shares something he has shared before, remember, he's human. So give him a great deal of grace, and double honor. Never murmur about him. If you don't like something he has said, pray about it, then leave the issue with God. If that doesn't satisfy you, leave the church, rather than divide it through murmuring and complaining.

A woman once spread some hot gossip about a local pastor. What he had supposedly done became common knowledge around town. Then she found that what she had heard wasn't true. She gallantly went to the pastor and asked for his forgiveness. The pastor forgave her, but then told her to take a pillow full of tiny feathers to a corner of the town, and in high winds, shake the feathers out. Then he told her to try to pick up every feather. He explained that the damage had already been done. She had destroyed his good reputation, and trying to repair the damage was like trying to pick up feathers in high winds.

The Bible says that there is life and death in the power of the tongue (Proverbs 18:21). We can kill or make something alive with our words. The Scriptures also reveal that God hates those who cause division among believers (Proverbs 6:16). Pray with the psalmist, "Set a guard, O LORD, over my mouth; keep watch over the door of my lips" (Psalm 141:3). Remember the old saying, "He who gossips *to* you, will gossip *about* you."

Thanksgiving—Do the Right Thing

For the Christian, every day should be Thanksgiving Day. We should be thankful even in the midst of problems. The apostle Paul said, "I am exceedingly joyful in all our tribulation" (2 Corinthians 7:4). He knew that God was working all things together for his good, even though he was going through trials (Romans 8:28). Problems *will* come your way. God will see to it personally that you grow as a Christian. He will allow storms in your life, in order to send your roots deep into the soil of His Word. We also pray more in the midst of problems. It's been well said that you will see more from your knees than on your tiptoes.

A man once watched a butterfly struggling to get out of its cocoon. In an effort to help it, he took a razor blade and carefully slit the edge of the cocoon. The butterfly escaped from its problem—and immediately died. It is God's way to have the butterfly struggle. It is the struggle that causes its tiny heart to beat fast and to send the life's blood into its wings. Trials have their purpose. They make us struggle—they bring us to our knees. They are the cocoon in which we often find ourselves.

It is there that the life blood of faith in God helps us spread our wings. Faith and thanksgiving are close friends. If you have faith in God, you will be thankful because you know His loving hand is upon you, even though you are in a lion's den. That will give you a deep sense of joy, and joy is the barometer of the depth of faith you have in God.

Let me give you an example. Imagine if I said I'd give you one million dollars if you sent me an email. Of course, you don't believe I would do that, but imagine if you did. Imagine if you knew 1,000 people who had sent me an email, and every one received their million dollars—no strings attached. More than that, you actually called me, and I assured you personally that I would keep my word. If you believed me, wouldn't you have joy? If you didn't believe me—no joy. The amount of joy you have would be a barometer of how much you believed my promise. We have so much for which to be thankful. God has given us "exceedingly great and precious promises" that are "more to be desired than gold." Do yourself a big favor: believe those promises, thank God continually for them, and "let your joy be full."

Water Baptism—Sprinkle or Immerse?

The Bible says, "Repent, and let every one of you be baptized in the name of Jesus

Christ for the remission of sins ..." (Acts 2:38). There is no question about whether you should be baptized. The questions are: How? When? And by whom? It would seem clear from Scripture that those who were baptized were fully immersed in water. Here's one reason:

> *"Now John also was baptizing in Aenon near Salim, because there was much water there" (John 3:23).*

If John were merely sprinkling believers, he would have needed only a cupful of water. Baptism by immersion pictures our death to sin, burial, and resurrection to new life in Christ (see Romans 6:4, Colossians 2:12). The Philippian jailer and his family were baptized at midnight, the same hour they believed. The Ethiopian eunuch was baptized as soon as he believed (Acts 8:35–37), as was Paul (Acts 9:17-18). Baptism is a step of obedience, and God blesses our obedience. So, what are you waiting for? Who should baptize you? It is clear from Scripture that other believers had the privilege, but check with your pastor, he may want the honor himself.

Giving—the Final Frontier

It has been said that the wallet is the "final frontier." It is the final area to be conquered—the last thing that we surrender to God. Jesus spoke much about money. He said that we cannot serve God and mammon (Matthew 6:24). The word "mammon" was the common Aramaic word for riches, which is related to a Hebrew word signifying "that which is to be trusted." In other words, we cannot trust God and money. Either money is our source of life, our great love, our joy, our sense of security, the supplier of our needs—or God is. When you open your purse or wallet, give generously and regularly to your local church. Whatever amount you give, make sure you give *something* to the work of God (see Malachi 3:8–10). Give because you want to, not because you have to. God loves a cheerful giver (2 Corinthians 9:7), so learn to hold your money with a loose hand.

Troubleshooting—Cults, Atheists, Skeptics

If you know the Lord, nothing will shake your faith. It is true that the man with an experience is not at the mercy of a man with an argument. If you are converted, and the

Holy Spirit "bears witness" that you are a child of God (Romans 8:16), you will never be shaken by a skeptic.

When cults tell you that you must acknowledge God's name to be saved, that you must worship on a certain day, or that you must be baptized by an elder of their church, don't panic. Merely go back to the Instruction Manual. The Bible has all the answers, and searching them out will make you grow. If you feel intimidated by atheists—if you think they are "intellectuals" —read my book *God Doesn't Believe in Atheists*. It will reveal that they are the opposite. It will also show you how to prove God's existence and also prove that the "atheist" doesn't exist.

Keep Fit

Finally, the way to prevent sporting injury and pain is to keep yourself fit. Exercise. The apostle Paul kept fit through exercise. He said, "Herein do I exercise myself, to always have a conscience void of offense toward God, and toward men" (Acts 24:16, KJV). Do the same. Listen to the voice of your conscience. It's your friend, not your enemy. Remember these words of Solomon:

> *"Fear God and keep His commandments, for this is the whole duty of man. For God will bring every work into judgment, including every secret thing, whether it is good or whether it is evil"* (Ecclesiastes 12:13,14).

Keep the Day of Judgment before your eyes. On that Day, you will be glad that you cultivated a tender conscience.

Your Prescription

I'm going to play "Doctor Comfort" for a moment. You are sick with fear. That is my diagnosis. Your disease is caused by the enemy of your soul. I am going to give you medicine that will heal you. The remedy to this disease is to take to heart the exceeding great and precious promises of God. (These have been placed in the Epilogue of this book.) Just as with a natural sickness, your doctor prescribes a medication and tells you to keep taking it *despite* persistent symptoms of your sickness, so it is with the spiritual sickness that plagues you. Discipline yourself to let these promises become a part of you. Take them. Absorb them into your system. Soak your soul in them. Renew your mind with them. Again, don't be concerned if you still have persistent symptoms of the disease; keep with the prescribed medicine. If symptoms persist, simply double the dose.

In *Pilgrim's Progress*, Christian and Faithful found themselves in Doubting Castle, being tormented by Giant Despair.[9] The situation was hopeless, until they found a way out of that fearful dungeon when Faithful put his hand into his breast and discovered the Key of Promise. Put these keys into your heart, and every time Giant Despair tries to lock you in his dirty dungeon of despair, take a firm grip of that liberating key. These are not ordinary promises. They are *supernatural*. They come from Almighty God Himself. The Bible says that He honors His Word above His name. So memorize them and then speak them out loud to the enemy whenever you detect his ugly presence.

The Bible says, "Submit to God. Resist the devil and he will flee from you." The key is first and foremost to be submitted to God (I trust that by now you are a fully armed Christian—that you have turned from sin and that your trust is in Jesus Christ), then resist the enemy with the Word of God.

The Bible calls the Word, "a two-edged sword" (see Ephesians 6:12-20). Take it out of its sheath and wield its flashing and fearsome blade. It shines with the very light of God Himself. He backs up every promise He has made. The enemy must bow to the Word of God. This is no exaggeration—a blind, anemic weak-kneed flea on crutches has infinitely more chance of defeating a herd of a thousand wild stampeding elephants than the devil has of defeating God.

So, do what Jesus did when the enemy came to torment Him, and tried to give Him suicidal thoughts. He *spoke* the Word of God to him (see Luke 4:5-10). I have heard demons scream in terror when Scripture was quoted[10] at them. (God is my witness that I'm speaking the truth.) So don't be passive. Be strong. Quote them with passion. Believe them with the utmost conviction. You are in a very real battle, so stand strong and tall, and fight with this most wonderful and powerful weapon.

I hope the principles I have shared with you have been helpful—that they are more than just comfort, and that, with the help of God, you find complete victory over panic attacks. If you know of someone who is suffering from irrational fear, please get this book into their hands.

May God bless you and keep you.

Epilogue

These are for you to copy and carry in your pocket and your heart.

The Promises of God (NKJV)

"I will not be afraid of ten thousands of people Who have set themselves against me all around" (Psalm 3:6).

"Though an army should encamp against me, My heart shall not fear; Though war should rise against me, In this I will be confident" (Psalm 27:3).

"Many are the afflictions of the righteous, But the Lord delivers him out of them all" (Psalm 34:19).

"You shall not be afraid of the terror by night, Nor of the arrow that flies by day" (Psalm 91:5).

"The Lord is on my side; I will not fear. What can man do to me?" (Psalm 118:6).

"When you lie down, you will not be afraid; yes, you will lie down and your sleep will be sweet. Do not be afraid of sudden terror, nor of trouble from the wicked when it comes; for the Lord will be your confidence, and will keep your foot from being caught" (Proverbs 3:24-26).

"When you pass through the waters, I will be with you; and through the rivers, they shall not overflow you. When you walk through the fire, you shall not be burned, nor shall the flame scorch you" (Isaiah 43:2).

"And we know that all things work together for good to those who love God, to those who are the called according to His purpose" (Romans 8:28).

"For our light affliction, which is but for a moment, is working for us a far more exceeding and eternal weight of glory, while we do not look at the things which are seen, but at the things which are not seen. For the things which are seen are temporary, but the things which are not seen are eternal" (2 Corinthians 4:17-18).

"Every word of God is pure; He is a shield to those who put their trust in Him" (Proverbs 30:5).

Comforting Promises

"It is of the Lord's mercies that we are not consumed, because His compassions fail not. They are new every morning: great is thy faithfulness ... For the Lord will not cast off forever: But though He cause grief, yet will He have compassion according to the multitude of His mercies. For He does not afflict willingly nor grieve the children of men" (Lamentations 3: 22-23, 31-32).

"Give ear to my prayer, O God; and hide not yourself from my supplication. Attend to me, and hear me: I mourn in my complaint, and make a noise; Because of the voice of the enemy, because of the oppression of the wicked: for they cast iniquity upon me, and in wrath they hate me. My heart is sore pained within me: and the terrors of death are fallen upon me. Fearfulness and trembling are come upon me, and horror has overwhelmed me. And I said, Oh that I had wings like a dove! for then would I fly away, and be at rest … As for me, I will call upon God; and the Lord shall save me. Evening, and morning, and at noon, will I pray, and cry aloud: and he shall hear my voice" (Psalm 55:1-6, 16-17).

Footnotes

1   The Bible says that God appreciates a broken (yielded) and contrite (repentant) spirit (see Psalm 51:17).

2   See Job chapter one.

3   See Acts chapters 8 & 9.

4   See job 2:6.

5   See *Spurgeon Gold* (Bridge-Logos Publishers).

6   Spurgeon, Charles, *Spurgeon's Sermons Volume 61*

7   Oswald Chambers: *Abandoned to God*

8   Ibid.

9   See *How To Win Souls and Influence People* by Ray Comfort (Bridge-Logos Publishers).

10 See *Out of the Comfort Zone* by Ray Comfort (Bridge-Logos Publishers).

"The Way of the Master"
Evidence Bible

Prove God's existence. Answer 100 common objections to Christianity. Show the Bible's supernatural origin. This unique study Bible includes wisdom from the foremost Christian leaders of yesterday and today such as Charles Spurgeon, D.L. Moody, John Wesley, Charles Finney, George Whitefield, Billy Graham, Dr. Bill Bright, John MacArthur, and R.C. Sproul.

Complete Bible available in
- Hardback
- Leather-bound (black or burgundy)
- Paperback

New Testament, Proverbs & Pslams available in
- Paperback
- Black leather-bound pocket editon

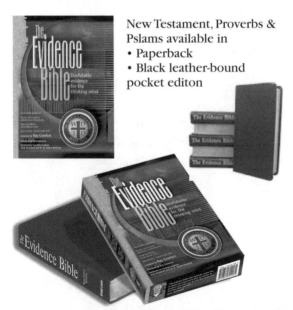

More **Bridge-Logos** Titles
from Ray Comfort

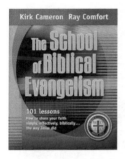

The School of Biblical Evangelism

In this comprehensive study course, you will learn how to share our faith simply, effectively, and biblically … the way Jesus did. Discover the God-given evangelistic tools that will enable you to confidently talk about the Savior.

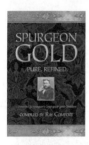

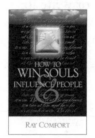

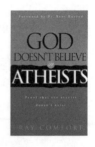

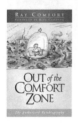

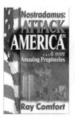

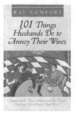

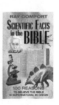

AVAILABLE AT FINE CHRISTIAN
BOOKSTORES

For More Information about Ray Comfort

visit www.livingwaters.com
call 1(800) 437-1893
or write to:
Living Waters Publications
P.O. Box 1172
Bellflower, CA 90706, USA